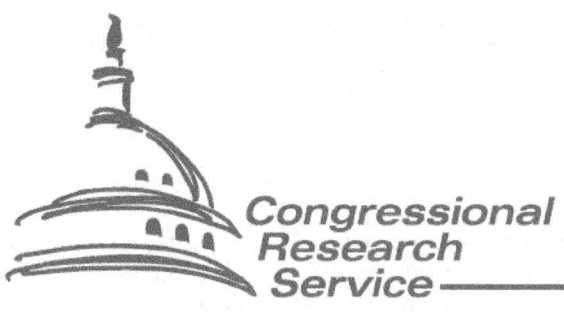

Congressional Research Service

Federal Employees Health Benefits Program (FEHBP): Available Health Insurance Options

Annie L. Mach
Analyst in Health Care Financing

Ada S. Cornell
Information Research Specialist

November 13, 2013

Congressional Research Service
7-5700
www.crs.gov
RS21974

CRS Report for Congress
Prepared for Members and Committees of Congress

Summary

FEHBP is generally available to federal employees, annuitants, and their dependents. Eligible individuals may elect coverage in an approved health benefits plan for either individual or family coverage. For the 2014 plan year, there are about 256 different plan choices, including all regionally available options. As a practical matter, an individual's choice of plans is often limited to 10 to 15 different plans, depending on where the individual resides. While enrollees have a range of choices, they typically decide which options best match their needs, the amount of their wages they will contribute to health insurance, and how risk-averse they are to potential out-of-pocket costs.

While most federal employees or annuitants reaching age 65 are automatically entitled to Medicare Part A, Medicare-eligible employees may also voluntarily choose to enroll in Medicare Part B and Part D. For individuals covered under a FEHBP plan as an annuitant, Medicare is the primary payer and FEHBP is the secondary payer. As a secondary payer, FEHBP could cover a share of Medicare deductibles and coinsurance for any services that are covered by both plans, and FEHBP would continue to reimburse for its covered services that are not covered by Medicare.

FEHBP is administered by the Office of Personnel Management (OPM), which is statutorily given the authority to contract with qualified carriers offering plans and to prescribe regulations necessary to carry out the statute, among other duties. Some of OPM's additional duties include coordinating the administration of FEHBP with employing offices, managing contingency reserve funds for the plans, and applying sanctions to health care providers according to the prescribed regulations.

Beginning in 2014, Members of Congress and certain congressional staff will no longer be eligible to enroll in a plan offered under FEHBP as an active employee; however, if they enroll in a health plan offered through a small business health option program (SHOP) exchange, they will remain eligible for an employer contribution toward coverage. For information about health benefits for Members and designated staff, please see CRS Report R43194, *Health Benefits for Members of Congress and Certain Congressional Staff*, by Annie L. Mach and Ada S. Cornell.

Contents

Figures

Tables

Appendixes

Contacts

FEHBP Basics

The statute governing the Federal Employees Health Benefits Program (FEHBP) is found in Title 5 of the U.S. Code, Chapter 89. The program is administered by the Office of Personnel Management (OPM), which is statutorily given the authority to contract with qualified carriers offering plans and to prescribe regulations necessary to carry out the statute, among other duties. (See **Appendix A** for a description of OPM's role in FEHBP.)

The federal government is the largest employer in the United States, and FEHBP is the largest employer-sponsored health insurance program. FEHBP covers about 8.2 million individuals, providing an estimated $47 billion annually in health care benefits. The participation rate among eligible enrollees is about 90% (85% of eligible individuals enroll in FEHBP as the primary policy holder, and another 5% are covered as a family member).[1]

Eligibility

Eligible enrollees include current federal employees, the President, annuitants, and eligible family members.[2] Active Members of Congress and certain congressional staff do not receive health benefits through FEHBP as a benefit of their employment, but may be eligible to enroll in FEHBP in retirement.[3] Newly hired employees have 60 days from their entry on duty date to sign up for an FEHBP plan.[4] Part-time workers are also eligible for coverage, but generally they are required to pay a larger share of premiums than full-time employees.[5]

In order to be eligible for FEHBP in retirement, an individual (1) must be entitled to retire on an immediate annuity under a retirement system for civilian employees (including FERS MRA + 10 retirements)[6] and (2) must have been continuously enrolled (or covered as a family member)

---

[1] OPM, "Fact Sheet: 2013 Federal Benefits Open Season for Health Benefits, Dental and Vision Insurance and Flexible Spending Accounts," available from OPM.

[2] Section 8901 of the FEHBP statute lists all of the eligibility groups, including for example, certain employees first employed by the government of the District of Columbia before October 1, 1987, among others. Additionally, eligibility information is provided in the *FEHB Program Handbook*, under "Eligibility for Health Benefits," http://www.opm.gov/healthcare-insurance/healthcare/reference-materials/reference/eligibility-for-health-benefits/.

[3] Section 1312(d)(3)(D) of the Patient Protection and Affordable Care Act (ACA, P.L. 111-148, as amended) requires that the only plans the federal government will be able to make available to Members of Congress and certain congressional staff will be those that are created under ACA or offered through an exchange. OPM issued a final rule that amends FEHBP eligibility to comply with Section 1312(d)(3)(D) of ACA on October 2, 2013 ("Federal Employees Health Benefits Program: Members of Congress and Congressional Staff," 78 *Federal Register* 60653, http://www.gpo.gov/fdsys/pkg/FR-2013-10-02/pdf/2013-23565.pdf). For more information about health benefits available to Members of Congress and certain congressional staff under ACA and the OPM final rule, see CRS Report R43194, *Health Benefits for Members of Congress and Certain Congressional Staff*, by Annie L. Mach and Ada S. Cornell.

[4] For newly hired employees, FEHBP coverage begins on the first day of the first pay period that begins after the employee's agency receives the employee's enrollment request.

[5] Certain temporary federal employees may also be eligible for FEHBP. For example, temporary employees who have completed one year of continuous service are eligible, and such employees pay the total premium amount. Additionally, in July 2012 OPM extended FEHBP eligibility to temporary federal firefighters (77 *Federal Register* 42417, July 19, 2012). For more information about coverage for temporary federal firefighters, see http://www.opm.gov/insure/health/firefighters/index.asp.

[6] A separating Federal Employees Retirement System (FERS) employee who is eligible for an immediate annuity under the minimum retirement age and 10 years of service (MRA + 10) provision may receive the benefits immediately or (continued...)

---

under FEHBP for the five years of service immediately before the date the annuity starts, or for the full period(s) of service since their first opportunity to enroll (if less than five years). The five-year requirement period can also include coverage under the Uniformed Services Health Benefits Program (also known as TRICARE) as long as the individual was covered under FEHBP at the time of retirement.[7]

Eligible family members include a spouse (or a valid common law marriage partner),[8] children under age 26, and continued coverage for qualified disabled children aged 26 years or older who are incapable of self-support because of a mental or physical disability that existed before age 26.[9] Under the Civil Service Retirement Spouse Equity Act of 1984, certain former spouses (of federal employees, former employees, and annuitants) may qualify to enroll in a health benefits plan under FEHBP.[10]

TRICARE and Civilian Health and Medical Program of the Department of Veterans Affairs (CHAMPVA) eligible FEHBP annuitants, survivors, and former spouses may suspend their FEHBP enrollment and then return to FEHBP during the open season, or return to FEHBP coverage immediately if they involuntarily lose this non-FEHBP coverage. Annuitants or former spouses who are enrolled in Medicare Parts A and B may suspend FEHBP enrollment to enroll in a Medicare Advantage plan (basically, a Medicare HMO or regional preferred provider organization [PPO]), with the option to re-enroll in FEHBP during open season, or sooner, if they involuntarily lose coverage or move out of the Medicare Advantage plan's service area.

Federal employee reservists who are placed in a leave without pay status when called to active duty for more than 30 days can keep their FEHBP coverage for up to 18 months. The reservist is responsible for paying the enrollee share of the premium during the first 12 months, and the agency pays the agency's share.

Since May 1, 2012, eligible Indian tribes, tribal organizations, and urban Indian organizations have been allowed to purchase FEHBP for their tribal employees.[11] The tribe or tribal

---

(...continued)

may postpone receiving an annuity to lessen the age reduction applicable to persons under age 62. If the individual is eligible for an MRA + 10 annuity and is not applying for the annuity at the time of separation, he or she may reenroll in FEHBP when the annuity begins. However, if the individual applies for an immediate annuity under the MRA + 10 provisions and later decides to postpone the annuity starting date he or she would not be able to enroll in FEHBP. Individuals retiring under the Civil Service Retirement System, who qualify for an immediate annuity, must retire on an immediate annuity and cannot postpone receiving the annuity (and therefore cannot postpone receiving FEHBP).

[7] OPM has the authority to waive the five-year requirement when it determines that it would be against equity and good conscience to not allow an annuitant to be enrolled in FEHBP (P.L. 99-251). For more information, see the *FEHB Program Handbook*, under "Annuitants and Compensationers," http://www.opm.gov/healthcare-insurance/healthcare/reference-materials/reference/annuitants-and-compensationers/.

[8] On June 26, 2013, the U.S. Supreme Court ruled that Section 3 of the Defense of Marriage Act (DOMA) is unconstitutional. As a result of the decision, OPM has stated that all legally married same-sex spouses are considered eligible family members under FEHBP. Additionally, the children (including step-children) of same-sex marriages are treated the same way as children of opposite-sex marriages for eligibility purposes. For more information, see http://www.opm.gov/healthcare-insurance/healthcare/carriers/2013/2013-20.pdf.

[9] For more information on children's eligibility up to age 26, see the Appendix of CRS Report R42741, *Laws Affecting the Federal Employees Health Benefits Program (FEHBP)*, by Annie L. Mach and Ada S. Cornell.

[10] For more information about the history of FEHBP eligibility, see the "Eligibility" section in CRS Report R42741, *Laws Affecting the Federal Employees Health Benefits Program (FEHBP)*, by Annie L. Mach and Ada S. Cornell.

[11] 25 U.S.C. §1647b.

---

organization is required to pay the government's share of the premium, at a minimum, with the enrollee paying the remaining share. Tribes and tribal organizations are only allowed to purchase this coverage for employees; coverage is not available to their annuitants.[12] Approximately 53 tribes with 10,000 tribal employees are currently enrolled.[13]

Finally, certain individuals may be eligible to temporarily continue their FEHBP coverage after their regular coverage ends, under Temporary Continuation Coverage (TCC). TCC is similar to COBRA[14] coverage offered to individuals in the private sector. Federal employees and family members who lose their FEHBP coverage because of a qualifying event, such as job loss (except for gross misconduct), may be eligible for TCC. TCC enrollees may initially enroll in any FEHBP plan and may also change plans during open season, but they must pay the full premium for the plan they select (that is, both the employee and government shares of the premium) plus a 2% administrative charge. In general, TCC coverage is available to separating employees and their families for up to 18 months after the date of separation. Children aging out of their parent's plan (at age 26) and former spouses can continue TCC for up to 36 months.

Election of Coverage and Plan Choices

FEHBP eligible persons may elect coverage in an approved health benefits plan through the "individual" or the "family" options. For the 2014 plan year, FEHBP offers enrollees a choice of 15 plan choices that are available government-wide (although four are only open to certain types of employees, e.g., State Department employees).[15] In total, there are 256 different plan choices, including all regionally available options. In addition, many plans offer a choice of a standard option, high option, and/or a high-deductible plan. As a practical matter, depending on where an enrollee resides, his or her choice of plans and options is limited to about 10 to 15 different plans. Plan details for all FEHBP plans are available on the website of the Office of Personnel Management (OPM)—http://www.opm.gov. Since 2007, those eligible for FEHBP (whether or not they are actually enrolled) are also eligible to enroll in the Federal Employee Dental and Vision Insurance Program (FEDVIP), which provides supplemental dental and vision insurance.

Plan Facts

Participation in FEHBP is voluntary, and enrollees may change plans during designated annual "open season" periods. Individuals who are eligible for, but not enrolled in, FEHBP may also enroll in a plan during open season. The open season for the 2014 plan year is from November 11 to December 9, 2013. Special enrollment periods are also allowed for those with a qualifying special circumstance, such as marriage. Enrollees are not subject to pre-existing condition exclusions.

---

[12] §157 of the Indian Health Care Improvement Reauthorization and Extension Act of 2009 (S. 1790) as enacted by §10221(a) of P.L. 111-148.

[13] OPM, "Fact Sheet: 2013 Federal Benefits Open Season for Health Benefits, Dental and Vision Insurance and Flexible Spending Accounts," available from OPM.

[14] For more information on COBRA, see CRS Report R40142, *Health Insurance Continuation Coverage Under COBRA*, by Janet Kinzer.

[15] OPM. Full Sets of Rate Charts. http://www.opm.gov/healthcare-insurance/healthcare/plan-information/premiums/.

Premiums

The government's share of premiums is set at 72% of the weighted average premium of all plans in the program, not to exceed 75% of any given plan's premium. The government's contribution to a plan for a part-time worker is generally prorated.[16] The maximum annual government contribution for 2013 is $5,114 for self-only coverage and $11,378 for family coverage.[17] The percentage of premiums paid by the government is calculated separately for individual and family coverage, but each uses the same formula. Annuitants and active employees pay the same premium amounts, although active employees have the option of paying premiums on a pre-tax basis. The enrollee's share of premiums will rise by an average of 4.4% in 2014, a larger increase than the 3.7% increase in 2013.[18] While some plans had no increases in premiums, others had double-digit premium increases. However, looking only at premium increases may not give a complete picture of plan changes from one year to the next, as plans may also make changes in benefits or cost-sharing.

Setting Premiums

With regard to setting premium rates, the statute governing FEHBP allows OPM to contract with carriers on either an experience-rated basis or a community-rated basis. The premiums for experience-rated FEHBP plans are based on the claims of the plan's federal enrollees. Experience-rating in FEHBP is retrospective, with gains and losses carried forward in the next year's premium.

Community-rated plans are those whose payment is based on a per member per month capitation rate. Community-rating in FEHBP is prospective, and it has several different forms. Traditional community-rated (TCR) plans set the same rates for all groups in a community, regardless of the health risks and characteristics of any specific group. Alternatively, community-rating by class allows for rate adjustments among groups based on the age and sex distribution of each group. Adjusted community-rating allows for the use of experience of a particular group to influence the premiums for that group.[19] Community-rated plans in FEHBP do not vary rates for enrollees based on the enrollees' characteristics; rather, community-rated plans use the various forms of community-rating to set a rate that considers some characteristics of its FEHBP enrollees but applies the same rate to all FEHBP enrollees.

All TCR community-rated plans in FEHBP use the similarly sized subscriber group (SSSG) method to set premiums. SSSGs are a carrier's two employer groups that have a subscriber

---

[16] Part-time workers (working 16 to 32 hours a week) hired on or after April 8, 1979, are entitled to a partial government contribution in proportion to the number of hours they are scheduled to work in a pay period. Part-time workers hired before April 8, 1979 who have continued to serve on a part-time basis without a break in service are eligible for the full government contribution. Additionally, part-time employees who work less than 16 hours or more than 32 hours per week are entitled to the full government contribution. The amount of the prorated government contribution for a part-time employee is the ratio of scheduled part-time work hours to full-time hours (usually 80 hours per biweekly pay period) multiplied by the government contribution for full-time employees enrolled in that plan. The part-time employee pays the difference between the total premium and the prorated government contribution.

[17] This is the maximum government contribution for non-postal employees and annuitants. For information about premiums for employees of the United States Postal Service, see **Appendix B**.

[18] OPM, "Average FEHBP Premiums in 2014 for Annuitants & Non-Postal Employees," available from OPM.

[19] OPM, *Carrier Handbook: Federal Employees Health Benefits Program*, March 2003, http://www.opm.gov/carrier/handbook/carrier_handbook.pdf.

---

enrollment closest in size to the FEHBP subscriber enrollment (as of the date specified by OPM in rate instructions); use any rating method other than retrospective experience-rating; and meet the criteria specified in the rate instructions by OPM. Using the SSSG method, the premiums of FEHBP TCR community-rated plans are compared to the premiums of SSSGs to ensure that FEHBP receives the lowest available premiums.

Previously, *non-TCR* community-rated plans in FEHBP also used the SSSG method to set premiums; however, beginning in plan year 2013, all non-TCR FEHBP community-rated plans must meet a FEHBP-specific medical loss ratio (MLR).[20] The 2014 FEHBP-specific MLR target is 85%.

An MLR is the ratio of plan incurred claims, including any expenditures that improve the quality of health care, to a plan's total premium revenue. The FEHBP-specific MLR is analogous to the MLR defined in the Patient Protection and Affordable Care Act (ACA, P.L. 111-148, as amended),[21] which FEHBP plans are also subject to.[22] However, the FEHBP MLR can be different from the ACA MLR, and all non-TCR community-rated FEHBP plans will be subject to both MLRs (all other FEHBP plans are only subject to the ACA MLR). FEHBP carriers will report the same categories of information for the FEHBP MLR as they do for the ACA MLR, but the FEHBP MLR calculation will only be based on the FEHBP population. Each year OPM will put forth the FEHBP MLR at least 12 months prior to the beginning of the plan year to which the MLR applies.

If a plan falls below the FEHBP MLR threshold, the plan must pay a subsidization penalty into a Subsidization Penalty Account. All plans will pay into the account and the funds will be annually distributed on a pro-rata basis to the contingency reserves of all non-TCR community-rated plans.

Benefits

Although there is no core or standard benefit package required for FEHBP, the statute requires that all plans cover basic hospital, surgical, physician, and emergency care. OPM may prescribe reasonable minimum standards for health benefit plans. FEHBP follows the guidelines on preventive care for children recommended by the American Academy of Pediatrics. FEHBP guidelines on preventive care for adults are based on accepted medical practice, and since 2011 all FEHBP plans have covered ACA-required preventive care services without imposing cost-sharing requirements.[23] OPM requires plans to cover certain special benefits including prescription drugs (which may have separate deductibles and coinsurance); mental health care

---

[20] 77 *Federal Register* 19522, April 2, 2012. TCR plans set the same rates for all groups in a community, regardless of the health risks and characteristics of any specific group. In TCR, healthier groups subsidize less healthy groups by design, and the TCR plans cannot adjust premiums for any specific group. Because of this, OPM believes it is inappropriate to impose the new rate-setting methodology on TCR plans. Currently, the only plans that use TCR are in states that require TCR.

[21] For more information about the ACA MLR, see CRS Report R42735, *Medical Loss Ratio Requirements Under the Patient Protection and Affordable Care Act (ACA): Issues for Congress*, by Suzanne M. Kirchhoff.

[22] The ACA MLR provision requires that health insurance issuers, beginning in 2011, meet an MLR of 85% for large group plans. For more information, see CRS Report R42735, *Medical Loss Ratio Requirements Under the Patient Protection and Affordable Care Act (ACA): Issues for Congress*, by Suzanne M. Kirchhoff.

[23] However, plans may choose to only waive cost-sharing when beneficiaries use in-network providers, so that if beneficiaries use out-of-network providers, they may still be responsible for cost-sharing under the terms and conditions of the plan.

---

with parity of coverage for mental health and general medical care coverage; child immunizations; and limits on an enrollee's total out-of-pocket costs for a year, called the catastrophic limit. Generally, once an enrollee's covered out-of-pocket expenditures reach the catastrophic limit, the plan pays 100% of covered medical expenses for the remainder of the year. Plans must also include certain cost-containment provisions, such as offering preferred provider organization (PPO) networks in fee-for-service plans and hospital pre-admission certification.

Additionally, since 2011, all plans offer tobacco cessation benefits in compliance with the U.S. Public Health Service's 2008 clinical guidance on tobacco cessation. Enrollees do not pay co-payments for the following benefits: (1) seven FDA-approved medications and (2) four counseling sessions per an attempt to quit smoking (with two covered attempts per year). Beginning in 2013, plans could choose (but were not required) to cover Applied Behavior Analysis (ABA) for children with autism.[24]

FEHBP Carriers

The law defines a FEHBP "carrier" to be a voluntary association, corporation, partnership, or other nongovernmental organization engaged in providing, paying for, or reimbursing the cost of health services, in consideration of premiums or other periodic charges payable to the carrier.[25] Each carrier contracts with OPM after a negotiation process that begins with OPM issuing its annual "call letter" asking for benefit and rate proposals.[26] Carrier contracts are at the legal entity level and not the parent organization. Therefore, a parent organization, such as Kaiser Permanente, may have multiple carrier organizations within FEHBP.[27] As illustrated in **Figure 1**, FEHBP enrollment is concentrated among a few parent organizations, with the vast majority of enrollment concentrated in the Blue Cross Blue Shield Association (BCBSA) plans.[28] Approximately 94% of all policy holders in FEHBP are enrolled in the top 10 parent organizations (by number of enrolled policy holders) shown in **Figure 1**.

---

[24] Previously, ABA was considered an educational intervention rather than a medical therapy, and it could not be covered under FEHBP.

[25] 5 USC §8901.

[26] OPM, "Federal Employees Health Benefits Program Call Letter," Letter No. 2013-04: March 21, 2013. http://www.opm.gov/healthcare-insurance/healthcare/carriers/2013/2013-04.pdf. See **Appendix A** for discussion of contract cycle and Annual Call Letters.

[27] A "parent organization" is a company that owns all or enough of another firm to control its management. The controlled firm is considered a subsidiary of the parent company. In some cases, the parent organization is the FEHBP carrier (e.g., GEHA). In other cases, the parent organization may have multiple FEHBP carriers. For example, Kaiser Permanente (KP) has the following subsidiary FEHBP carriers: KP of Georgia, KP of Colorado, KP of Hawaii, KP Mid-Atlantic, KP of Northern California, KP Northwest, KP of Southern California, and KP of Ohio.

[28] The Blue Cross Blue Shield Association (BCBSA) includes both the nonprofit national carriers operated by the BCBSA and the nonprofit local carriers typically organized at the state level. BCBSA does not include the for-profit WellPoint-Anthem carriers that use the Blue Cross Blue Shield marketing name. Approximately 96% of all individuals enrolled in the BCBSA plans are enrolled in plans offered by the nonprofit national carriers.

Figure 1. Top 10 Parent Organizations, by Covered Policy Holders, 2013

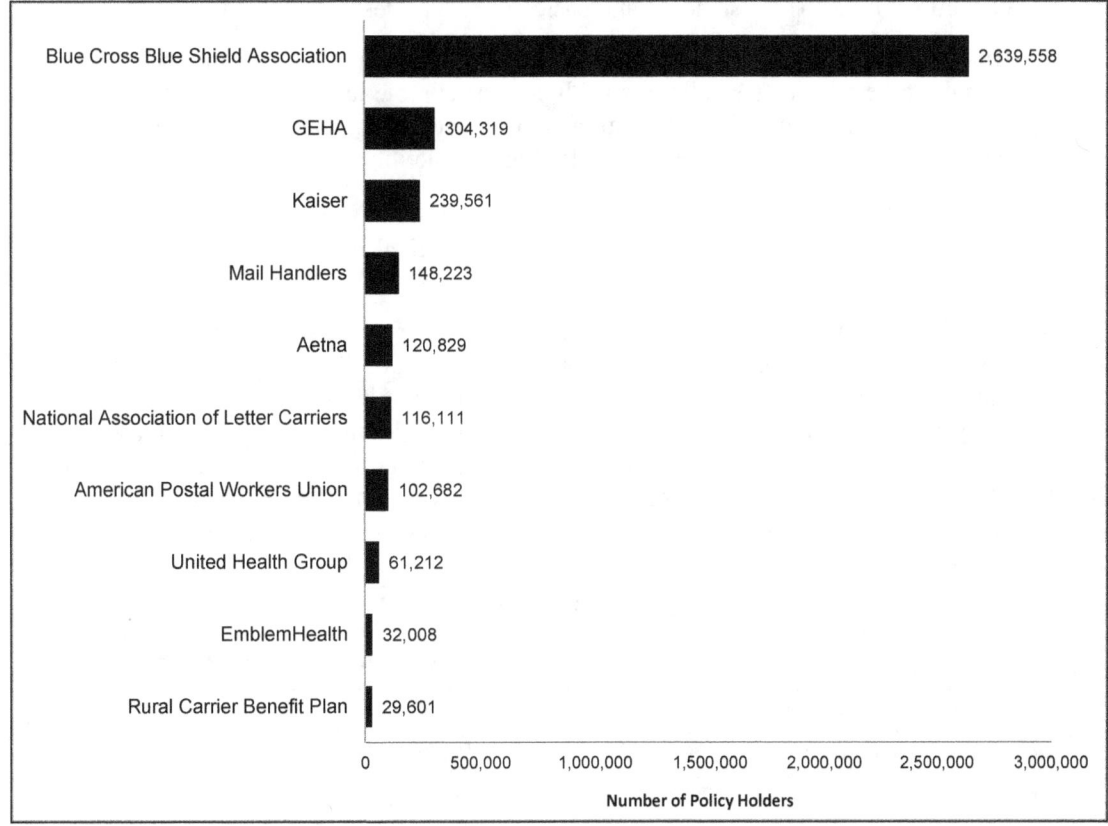

Source: CRS analysis of "FEHBP OPM Headcount Totals for 2013" data from OPM.

Notes: The numbers in this figure represent enrollment of policy holders; the numbers do not include enrollment of dependents.

The Blue Cross Blue Shield Association (BCBSA) includes both the nonprofit national carriers operated by the BCBSA and the nonprofit local carriers typically organized at the state level. BCBSA does not include the for-profit WellPoint-Anthem carriers that use the Blue Cross Blue Shield marketing name. Approximately 96% of all individuals enrolled in BCBSA plans are enrolled in the plans offered by the nonprofit national carriers.

FEHBP Plans

An FEHBP health benefits plan is a group insurance policy or similar group arrangement provided by a carrier to provide, pay for, or reimburse expenses for health services. The FEHBP statute[29] specifies three types of participating plans that are currently offered:[30]

- The **government-wide service benefit plan** is the fee-for-service benefit plan that pays providers directly for services (this slot has always been filled by Blue

---

[29] 5 USC §8903.

[30] The statute also specifies that OPM may contract with an indemnity benefit plan, which is a government-wide plan offering two levels of benefits. Aetna offered the indemnity benefit plan under FEHBP from the program's creation through 1989. Since then, OPM has not contracted with an insurer to offer the indemnity benefit plan.

Cross and Blue Shield, BCBS).[31] As of 2010, BCBS no longer offers a high-deductible plan, just the standard and basic options, as described below.

- **Employee organization plans** are fee-for-service plans, such as the American Postal Workers Union (APWU) plan. All persons eligible to enroll in FEHBP may choose any employee organization plan, subject to small annual membership dues. These plans also include options for high-deductible plans.

- **Comprehensive medical plans** are the local Health Maintenance Organizations (HMOs). Availability of these plans varies, depending on where the individual resides. These plans also include options for high-deductible plans.

Deductibles, copayments, and coinsurance amounts vary across plans. Many plans offer two or more options with different premiums and levels of coverage. Even within individual plans, enrollees are offered a lower deductible and coinsurance amount if they choose to use services, such as a physician or hospital provider, in the plan's network. Examining the premiums, deductibles, copayment, and coinsurance amounts for physician office visits in the Blue Cross and Blue Shield (BCBS) plans provides an example of this variation (See **Table 1**). For 2014, BCBS offers both a *Standard* option (its more generous plan) and a *Basic* option.

Table 1. Standard and Basic BCBS Plans, 2014

	BCBS Standard Option	BCBS Basic Option
Premiums – Individual Coverage		
Enrollee's share of monthly premium amount	$190.28	$132.09
Percent change in enrollee's contribution, 2013 to 2014	+2.2%	+3.2%
Premiums – Family Coverage		
Enrollee's share of monthly premium amount	$444.12	$309.30
Percent change in enrollee's contribution, 2013 to 2014	+2.4%	+3.2%
Cost-sharing – Both Types of Coverage		
Calendar year deductible	$350 per person; $700 per family	None
Copayment for preferred primary care provider office visit	$20[a]	$25
Copayment for preferred specialist office visit	$30[a]	$35
Coinsurance for participating provider visit	35% of plan allowance	N/A[b]
Coinsurance for nonparticipating provider visit	35% of plan allowance, plus any difference between allowance and billed amount	N/A[b]

---

[31] The Blue Cross Blue Shield (BCBS) plan that occupies this slot is the nonprofit national carrier; the nonprofit local carriers that operate under the Blue Cross Blue Shield Association (BCBSA) are not considered government-wide service benefit plans. For more information about the BCBSA, see http://www.bcbs.com/about-the-association/.

Source: Blue Cross® and Blue Shield ® Service Benefit Plan, 2014. http://www.fepblue.org/downloads/2014_SBP_BROCHURE_20141243.pdf.

a.   The calendar year deductible does not apply for this benefit.

b.   The Basic option operates similarly to an HMO, in that enrollees may use only preferred providers to receive benefits, except in special circumstances such as emergency care.

High-Deductible Plans Combined with Tax-Advantaged Accounts

In 2003, FEHBP began offering high-deductible plans coupled with tax-advantaged accounts that could be used to pay for qualified medical expenses. These plans are believed to help control costs by exposing enrollees to more risk for their health care expenditures. FEHBP first offered this arrangement by combining a consumer-driven health plan (CDHP) with a Health Reimbursement Arrangement (HRA). In 2005, FEHBP expanded this option to include a high-deductible health plan (HDHP) with either a Health Savings Account (HSA) or an HRA. Both the employee organization plans and the comprehensive medical plans offer CDHPs and HDHPs, described below.

Consumer-Driven Health Plans

For example, those choosing APWU's CDHP 2014 plan are provided with an HRA (referred to as a Personal Care Account, or PCA, in the APWU plan), which the plan funds in the amount of $1,200 for individuals and $2,400 for families. PCA funds are not taxable. Unused balances of a PCA may be carried over, with a limit of $5,000 for individuals and $10,000 for families, but balances are forfeited when an enrollee leaves the plan.[32]

In APWU's CDHP, all eligible health care expenses (except in-network preventive care) are paid first from the PCA. Eligible expenses include basic medical, surgical hospital, prescription drug and other services covered under the high-deductible plan, as well as dental and vision services (with a limit of up to $400 per year for self and $800 for family). Once the enrollee has spent the annual amount contributed by the plan to the PCA (i.e., $1,200 or $2,400), enrollees must pay the deductible for the traditional health coverage ($600 for individuals and $1,200 for families). Members who have exhausted their PCA must use their own funds to pay the deductible. However, members who have built up the balances in their PCA over time may use any excess funds to meet their deductible.[33] Once the deductible has been satisfied, the plan starts covering services, with copayments and coinsurance amounts similar to those found in traditional health plans.

Enrollee monthly premiums in 2014 increased 3% over 2013 rates to $97.42 for individual coverage and $219.15 for family coverage. While enrollees may use either in- or out-of-network providers, the PCA funds will go further for in-network providers. For example, amounts over the plan allowance for out-of-network services do not count toward reducing the deductible.

---

[32] APWU Health Plan, 2014. http://www.apwuhp.com/upload/2014_brochure.pdf.

[33] For example, for individual coverage, if the PCA balance is $2,000, the individual could use $1,200 from the fund to pay for services and another $600 from the fund to meet the deductible. The enrollee would then qualify for coverage under the health care plan while still retaining a PCA balance of $200.

In 2014, in addition to APWU's nationally available CDHP, two other plans, Aetna and Humana, also offer a CDHP. Although widely available, neither of these plans is nationally available. While these three plans are similar in many ways, there are some significant differences, including (1) the amount the plans place in the HRA, (2) the carryover amount, (3) rules for when the plan begins to cover medical expenses, (4) the catastrophic limit amount, and (5) availability. For example, Aetna's Medical Fund (similar to the PCA) is funded by the plan in the amount of $1,000 for individuals and $2,000 for families with no limits on carryover amounts, provided the enrollee remains in the plan.[34]

High-Deductible Plans with an HSA or HRA

Since 2005, FEHBP has offered several HDHP plans paired with either an HSA[35] or HRA, available both nationally and regionally for 2014. FEHBP's HRAs coupled with the HDHP are similar to HRAs offered with CDHPs, in that they (1) cannot exclude FEHBP-eligible individuals, (2) can only be used for medical expenses, (3) are not subject to tax, (4) are funded solely by the plan, (5) do not earn interest, and (6) are forfeited when an enrollee leaves the plan.

The rules for FEHBP HSAs coupled with an HDHP are very different. HSAs are only available to certain individuals: those who are not enrolled in Medicare, not covered by another health plan, not claimed as a dependent on someone else's federal tax return, and those who have not received Department of Veterans Affairs health benefits in the past three months. Enrollees may add additional funds to their HSA, as long as the plan's and the enrollee's combined contributions do not exceed the federal limit (for 2014, the limit is $3,300 for self-coverage and $6,550 for family coverage).[36] Enrollees from ages 55 up to age 65 can make a "catch-up" contribution of up to $1,000.[37] The plan's contribution to the HSA is tax-free, an enrollee's contribution is tax-deductible (an above-the line deduction, not limited to those who itemize), and any interest earned is tax-free. All unused funds, as well any interest, may be carried over each year without limit. In addition to qualified medical expenses, in 2014, HSA funds may also be used for nonmedical expenses, subject to the income tax and an additional penalty for those under 65.[38] Each month, the plan automatically deposits a portion of the FEHBP HDHP premiums into an HSA or HRA. Individuals enrolled in an HDHP who are not eligible for an HSA, as of the first day of the month, have their funds credited to an HRA. Plans place the same amount into an enrollee's HRA as they do into an HSA.

Examining GEHA's HDHP provides an example of premiums, deductibles and HSA/HRAs for these types of plans. For individual coverage in 2014, the employee's share of the monthly premium is $110.21, the deductible is $1,500, the plan will place $62.50 per month in the HSA/HRA, and those in the HSA may contribute another $2,550 annually (the difference

---

[34] Aetna HealthFund® CDHP / Aetna Value Plan, 2014. http://www.aetnafeds.com/pdf/2014/2014CDHPValueBrochure.pdf.

[35] For more information on HSAs, see CRS Report RS21573, *Tax-Advantaged Accounts for Health Care Expenses: Side-by-Side Comparison, 2013*, by Carol Rapaport.

[36] IRS. Rev. Proc. 2013-25. http://www.irs.gov/pub/irs-drop/rp-13-25.pdf.

[37] OPM. "Comparison Chart for Health Savings Account, Health Reimbursement Arrangement, Health Care Flexible Spending Account, and Limited Expense Health Care Flexible Spending Account," http://www.opm.gov/healthcare-insurance/healthcare/health-savings-accounts/comparison-chart/.

[38] ACA raised the penalty from 10% to 20% for those under 65 who make a nonqualified withdrawal from an HSA, beginning in 2011.

between the amount contributed by the plan and the federal self-coverage limit). For family coverage in 2014, the employee's share of the monthly premium is $251.72; the deductible is $3,000; the plan places $125 per month into the HSA/HRA;[39] and those with an HSA may contribute another $5,050 annually (the difference between the amount contributed by the plan and the federal family coverage limit). Enrollees over age 55 may also make "catch-up" contributions. For 2014, GEHA's HDHP premiums increased 5% for individual coverage and family coverage from the 2013 amounts. Neither deductibles nor annual HSA/HRA contributions made by the plan changed from the 2013 amounts.[40]

Flexible Spending Accounts and Their Role in FEHBP

Active federal employees (not annuitants) may participate in the federal Flexible Spending Accounts (FSA) program, consisting of a Health Care FSA and a Dependent Care FSA.[41] Contributions to an FSA are voluntary, with accounts funded solely by an employee from his or her pre-taxed salary, thereby reducing taxable income. The government does not make any contribution to the FSA. Funds in a Health Care FSA (HCFSA) can be used to pay for qualified medical expenses that are not reimbursed or covered by any other source. Qualified medical expenses include coinsurance amounts, copayments, deductibles, dental care, glasses, and hearing aids.[42]

Employees choosing to participate in an HCFSA must contribute at least $250 and no more than $2,500 per year to an account,[43] and the total pledged contribution for the year is available at the start of the year. HCFSA funds can be carried over for 2½ months after the end of the plan year (for example, 2013 contributions to the HCFSA may be used to reimburse expenses incurred during calendar year 2013 continuing through mid-March 2014); unused funds are forfeited.[44] During the annual FEHBP open season, employees may voluntarily make an election for an HCFSA amount to be set aside in the upcoming year. Employees eligible for FEHBP (even those not currently enrolled) may elect an HCFSA. Under Internal Revenue Code rules, only current employees—not annuitants—are eligible to contribute to an HCFSA.

---

[39] For 2014, the HRA annual credit is $750 (prorated for mid-year enrollment).

[40] Government Employees Health Association (GEHA), 2014 Health Savings Advantage HDHP Brochure, https://www.geha.com/FAQs-and-Resources/Form-and-Document-Library/Health-Savings-Advantage-HDHP/2014-Health-Savings-Advantage-HDHP-Brochure.

[41] For more information on FSAs, see CRS Report RS21573, *Tax-Advantaged Accounts for Health Care Expenses: Side-by-Side Comparison, 2013*, by Carol Rapaport.

[42] The ACA changed the definition of qualified medical expenses, beginning in 2011. The ACA does not allow over-the-counter (OTC) medicines to be covered by these tax-advantaged accounts unless they are prescribed by a physician, with the exception of insulin. Other currently eligible OTC items that are not medicines or drugs, such as bandages, will not require a prescription. The FSA program provides a complete list of covered and noncovered medical expenses: http://www fsafeds.com.

[43] The ACA established a contribution limit of $2,500 for FSAs, beginning in 2013. In subsequent years the threshold is indexed to inflation, but it remained unchanged in 2014. Prior to 2013 the maximum annual contribution amount was $5,000.

[44] The Department of Treasury and Internal Revenue Service (IRS) recently issued Notice 2013-71, which modifies the "use it or lose it" aspect of FSAs. The guidance indicates that employers may choose whether to offer their employees the 2½ month grace period or allow their employees to carryover up to $500 of unused amounts into the next plan year. As of the date of this report, OPM has not indicated whether it will modify the HCFSA arrangement from allowing a grace period to allowing employees to carryover funds. For more information about the modification, see http://www.irs.gov/pub/irs-drop/n-13-71.pdf.

Individuals who are enrolled in either a CDHP or HDHP coupled with an HRA may also enroll in the HCFSA, as long as they are not annuitants. Individuals enrolled in an HSA may also enroll in a limited expense HCFSA (LEX HCFSA) that can be used to cover qualified dental and vision care. Individuals may weigh the pros and cons of the LEX HCFSA coupled with an HSA against a standard HCFSA, choosing the one that best fits their needs, especially if they have a large expense that can only be covered by the standard HCFSA, such as a hearing aid. On the other hand, HSA funds can be carried over from year to year, and some of the funding in the HSA comes from the plan.

Medicare and FEHBP

Most federal employees or annuitants reaching age 65 are automatically entitled to premium-free Part A of Medicare, Hospital Insurance (HI), because they or their spouse paid Medicare payroll taxes for at least 40 quarters (10 years). Federal workers and their employer each pay 1.45% of earnings for Medicare payroll taxes. Medicare Part B Supplementary Medicare Insurance (SMI) and Part D prescription drug coverage are voluntary, and qualified individuals choosing to enroll must pay a monthly premium. Generally, individuals who do not enroll in Parts B or D during their initial eligibility period are subject to a penalty if they enroll at a later date. However, for Part B, individuals covered by an FEHBP plan either through their own or a spouse's active employment (not annuitant coverage) may wait until either they or their spouse retires to enroll without incurring a delayed enrollment penalty. Upon retirement, individuals must enroll in Part B or be subject to a late enrollment penalty if they enroll at a later date. For Part D, the prescription drug coverage included in FEHBP plans is determined to be at least actuarially equivalent to Part D, on average. Therefore, if an individual maintains FEHBP coverage and at a later date decides to enroll in Part D, there is no late enrollment penalty.[45] Annuitants or former spouses enrolled in Medicare Parts A and B may suspend FEHBP enrollment to enroll in a Medicare Advantage plan (e.g., a Medicare HMO or regional PPO), with the option to re-enroll in FEHBP during open season, or sooner, if they involuntarily lose coverage or move out of the Medicare Advantage plan's service area.

For individuals who are covered under an FEHBP plan through annuitant coverage (not active employment), any Medicare coverage they have would be the primary payer and FEHBP would be the secondary payer. As the secondary payer, FEHBP could cover a share of Medicare deductibles and coinsurance for any services that were covered by both Medicare and the plan. Enrollees may have to pay a share of the cost-sharing or deductibles. Additionally, the plan would continue to provide reimbursement for its covered services that were not covered by Medicare.

For retirees (or spouses) over the age of 65 who do not have either Medicare Parts A or B or both, FEHBP plans are the primary payer, and the plan pays hospitals and physicians based upon Medicare rates. For these individuals, the FEHBP benefit payment for inpatient hospital services is equivalent to the Medicare payment (the amount of the payment before the Medicare deductible, coinsurance, and lifetime limits are applied), reduced by any FEHBP deductible, coinsurance, copayment, or readmission certification penalty. For these individuals, the FEHBP payment for physician services is the lower of the Medicare Part B payment or the actual billed charges. The payment is then reduced by any FEHBP deductible, coinsurance, or copayment that

---

[45] The same rules for Medicare late enrollment penalties also apply to those with coverage through a private-sector employer.

is the responsibility of the retired individual. Hospitals may not collect, from either FEHBP or enrollees, more than the amount determined to be equivalent to the Medicare payment. For physician services, (1) Medicare participating providers may not collect from either FEHBP or Medicare-eligible enrollees more than the total Medicare payment under the Medicare participating physician fee schedule, and (2) Medicare nonparticipating providers may not collect from FEHBP plans or Medicare-eligible enrollees more than the Medicare limiting charge amount. (Under Medicare, nonparticipating physicians can balance bill up to 15% higher than the fee schedule amount, but they are paid a slightly lower amount by Medicare.)

Affordable Care Act and FEHBP

FEHBP plans must comply with a number of ACA provisions. Some ACA provisions have no meaningful effect on FEHBP as the plans already meet the requirements of the provision, while other provisions confer new requirements on the plans. OPM has provided FEHBP plans with guidance on how to implement ACA provisions; in some cases, OPM has expanded the scope of ACA provisions. For example, OPM requires FEHBP plans to implement some ACA provisions prior to their effective dates as specified in ACA. For a detailed list of ACA provisions that affect FEHBP, see CRS Report R42741, *Laws Affecting the Federal Employees Health Benefits Program (FEHBP)*, by Annie L. Mach and Ada S. Cornell.

Conclusion

FEHBP's wide range of options allows enrollees to use their own authority to hold down their health insurance costs, and because premiums are based on an average of all plan costs, individual decisions ultimately affect all enrollees. Eligible enrollees typically weigh personal factors, such as how much of their wages they are willing to contribute to health insurance and how risk-averse they are to potential out-of-pocket costs. FEHBP-eligible individuals may revisit their decision every year during the annual open season. Individuals who find themselves with too much or too little risk, under- or over-coverage, and those whose health status changes, may change plans each year. In the past, there has been little movement from one plan to another each year. More than one-half of all FEHBP-eligible individuals are enrolled in a Blue Cross and Blue Shield plan, and even those enrolled in other FEHBP plans tend to remain in their plan from year to year.

Appendix A. OPM's Role in FEHBP

FEHBP is offered under the authority of statute (Chapter 89 of title 5 of the U.S. Code) and is administered by the Office of Personnel Management (OPM) in accordance with the statute and its implementing regulations (5 CFR Part 89, and 48 CFR Chapter 16). The FEHBP statute establishes the basic rules for benefits, enrollment, and participation in FEHBP among other general requirements, while still allowing OPM wide authority in implementing regulations, contracting with plans, establishing benefits, and administering FEHBP.

In general, OPM, the employing offices of agencies (such as the Department of Labor), and the plans, each have defined roles in FEHBP. OPM is authorized to contract with insurance carriers; approve qualified health benefits plans for participation in the program; negotiate with plans about benefit and premium levels; determine the times and conditions for open seasons during which eligible individuals may elect coverage or change plans; make information available to employees concerning plan options; apply administrative sanctions to health care providers who have committed certain violations; and administer the financing of the program. OPM is responsible for maintaining the funds that hold contingency reserves for the plans and the fund that receives premium payments from enrollees and employing agencies, from which premiums are disbursed to participating plans.

OPM supervises all health insurance activities for annuitants. OPM determines whether retiring employees or survivor annuitants meet the requirements to continue health insurance coverage; takes the action necessary to terminate, accept, or continue enrollment; oversees the automatic deduction of premiums from monthly annuity checks and credits the premiums, along with the applicable government contribution, to the proper account; processes all enrollment changes; notifies affected carriers of enrollment changes; and keeps enrolled annuitants advised of rate and benefit changes within their plan.

The employing offices manage FEHBP for their employees according to OPM requirements, administer open season, and are responsible for payroll withholdings and the government contribution. The plans process and pay claims, print brochures according to OPM specifications, and maintain data on enrollment, claims, and financial information. Plans assume the risk for covering claims.

Annual Cycle of FEHBP Activity for OPM

OPM enters into an annual contract with carriers, following the negotiation process. Each spring, the annual negotiation process begins when OPM sends all current and newly approved qualified health plans an annual call letter to advise them on goals and procedures for negotiating contracts for the following calendar year and to request participating plans to submit their benefit and rate proposals for the next year. The call letter includes any changes in the services OPM seeks to make available for federal workers and annuitants, as well as notification of services that OPM discourages.

Next, OPM reviews proposals for rates (premiums) for the fee-for-service plans in relation to many factors, including the cost of covered services, managed care initiatives, the plan's past experience, health care utilization patterns of the enrolled group, and health care cost inflation in general. Pursuant to the negotiations, OPM and the plans (including both fee-for-service plans and HMOs) agree to specific terms and conditions each party is obligated to meet in the next contract year. Descriptions of both covered and excluded services are incorporated into the final contracts, and the plans print brochures describing the benefits and costs according to a standard format specified by OPM. The brochures are binding statements of benefits and exclusions that plans must follow as parties to FEHBP contracts. OPM then announces an open season (which generally runs for one month, beginning in early November).

OPM prints and distributes to personnel offices and annuitants a guide describing the major features and premiums for all participating plans. This guide includes the findings of surveys of enrollee satisfaction with the different plans and includes information about the factors participants should consider in making their selection. Personal advice is not provided, although OPM's Internet website provides information about how to select a plan (http://www.opm.gov/insure). Employees are responsible for obtaining from their personnel office a copy of OPM's general guide and the detailed brochures of the specific plans in which they are interested. Annuitants are responsible for obtaining detailed plan brochures by calling the individual carriers and requesting that a brochure be mailed to them. Information about the different plans is also available on OPM's web page, http://www.opm.gov/insure.

Following is a summary of the annual cycle of OPM's activities regarding plan contracts:

- End of March/early April—Call letter distributed to plans
- May 31—Plan responses due to OPM (electronic format)
- June through August—Contract negotiations
- September/October—Print and distribute OPM guides and plan brochures
- November/December—Open season
- Early December/January 1—Enrollment data distributed to plans
- Early January—Plan year starts
- March—Reconciliation of HMO premiums

OPM's Annual Call Letters

Each spring, OPM issues a carrier letter to plans detailing the annual call for benefit and rate proposals from FEHBP carriers and outlining its policy goals for the following calendar year. It is not unusual for OPM to require that plans not increase premiums to cover the costs of new benefits; however, there are exceptions to this limitation. One exception may occur when OPM requires plans to offer a new benefit, such as the requirements to offer mental health parity for out-of-network benefits in compliance with Subtitle B of *Emergency Economic Stabilization Act of 2008*, entitled the "Paul Wellstone and Pete Domenici Mental Health Parity and Addiction Equity Act of 2008."

Another example of OPM using its authority is the requirement that all plans include coverage of prescription drugs, as first detailed in the annual call letter for the 1990 contract year. That letter stated:

> We believe at least minimum coverage for prescription drugs should be provided in all FEHBP plans (both options if plan has more than one), as it is for hospital and medical expense. We consider a minimum drug benefit as one with a deductible no greater than $600

and coinsurance of at least 50%.... Our decision on a mandatory minimum drug benefit will be communicated to you during the negotiations.[46]

Subsequent annual call letters have expanded and modified OPM's prescription drug requirements for plans.

OPM's Role with Employing Offices

Personnel offices in every federal agency manage participation in FEHBP for their employees according to procedures prescribed by OPM. They administer the annual open seasons; adjust coverage and payroll withholding when workers' family or employment situations change and when new workers enter. Agencies are responsible for withholding employee premium payments, adding the government's share (which is appropriated to agencies annually), and providing documentation of these actions to OPM. They keep records and information on withholdings from employee salaries and agency contributions, enrollment statistics, and other necessary data.

The government's share of active workers' FEHBP premiums is paid by the government agency for which the employee works. The money for agency payments is appropriated annually to every agency's salary and expense accounts, and, for federal budget purposes, is categorized as discretionary spending. The government's share of nonpostal annuitants' premiums is appropriated annually to OPM and is categorized in the federal budget as direct, or mandatory spending. The government's share of premiums for all nonpostal enrollees is paid from general revenues. The U.S. Postal Service (USPS) pays the employer share of FEHBP premiums for its workers and annuitants with funds taken in by the USPS from postal rate receipts, although the postal unions and the USPS collectively bargain the cost-sharing ratio for active workers.[47]

OPM's Role with the Plans

FEHBP plans are required to allow eligible individuals to enroll during open season and other special election periods and may not discriminate on the basis of health status, race, sex or age.[48] The carriers process and pay claims, answer enrollee questions, respond to claims disputes, print annual open season brochures according to the OPM-specified format, and maintain data regarding enrollment, claims, and other financial information required by OPM. In addition, carriers assume all insurance risk.

Contracts: The contracts OPM makes with FEHBP plans are made for at least one year and may be made automatically renewable in the absence of notice by either party of intention to terminate. OPM may terminate the contract of a carrier at the end of the year, if at no time during the preceding two contract terms did the carrier have 300 or more enrolled employees and annuitants, exclusive of family members. Each contract must contain a detailed statement of benefits. Contracts must offer enrollees and their family members temporary extension of coverage with an option to convert to a nongroup contract, without requiring evidence of good

---

[46] FEHB Program Carrier Letter, March 30, 1989.

[47] In FY2009 the USPS contribution to premiums was, on average, 81% of premiums while other federal government agencies paid, on average, 72% of premiums.

[48] 5 CFR §890.201.

health. Plans that are discontinued, other than through a merger, may re-enter after three contract years from the time they left the program.

Licensure: An FEHBP plan must be licensed to sell group health insurance under state law in every area of a state in which it operates as an FEHBP plan. Nationwide plans must be licensed in every state. HMOs must have an internal quality assurance program, and must credential and periodically re-credential participating providers. OPM requires that each FEHBP plan submit copies of its state license(s) with its application to participate in FEHBP; in addition, as part of the plan's contract with FEHBP the plan is required to inform OPM if a state has withdrawn, or intends to withdraw, the plan's license.

Quality: Each year FEHBP plans with 500 or more subscribers must mail the Consumers Assessment of Health Plan Survey (CAHPS) to a random sample of plan members. For HMOs, and Point-of-Service (POS) plans, the sample includes all commercial plan members, including nonfederal members. For Fee-for-Service (FFS)/Preferred Provider Organization (PPO) plans, the sample includes federal members only. The CAHPS survey consists of a set of standardized health plan performance measures that evaluate members' satisfaction with their health plans. Independent vendors certified by the National Committee for Quality Assurance (NCQA) administer the surveys. OPM sets CAHPS requirements for the plans each year, which include instructions to send OPM a copy of any survey results.

All plans must also complete quality assurance reports as well as fraud and abuse case reports and submit the reports to OPM. Additionally, HMOs with more than 500 FEHBP enrollees must complete the Health Plan and Employer Data Information Set (HEDIS), which includes clinical performance measures based on information such as members' medical records. Each year OPM outlines the procedures for collecting the HEDIS measures; these measures help to compare how well plans prevent and treat illness.

Provider Networks: OPM reviews applications for health benefit plans for evidence of a plan's ability to provide reasonable access to and choice of quality primary and specialty medical care throughout the service area, specifically (1) in the individual practice setting, contractual arrangements for the services of a significant number of primary care and specialty physicians in the service area; and (2) in the group practice setting, compliance with statutes, preferably demonstrated by full-time providers specializing in internal medicine, family practice, pediatrics, and obstetrics/gynecology.

OPM's Role with the Reserve Funds

A contingency reserve fund is maintained in the U.S. Treasury by OPM for all FEHBP plans. OPM is authorized to levy a surcharge of up to 3% of a plan's premium to establish and maintain contingency reserves.[49] The preferred minimum for each experience-rated plan's contingency reserve[50] is 1½ times the sum of the plan's average month's paid claims plus the average month's

---

[49] 5 CFR §890.503.

[50] All fee-for-service plans (and a small number of comprehensive plans) are "experience-rated," meaning the premiums are based on the claims experience of the federal enrollees in the plan in preceding years. Experience-rate plan premiums are based on claim experience of enrollees in previous years, administrative costs, and profit (limited to 1.1% of claims and administrative costs). There is little risk because they make up for losses with premium increases the following year or by drawing down on contingency reserve.

administrative expenses and retention. Experience-rated plans may use their contingency reserve funds to offset larger than anticipated claims, or, if the fund balance becomes larger than necessary, it can be drawn down and used to offset a premium increase in the subsequent year. Since January 1989, FEHBP fee-for-service plans have had their federal premium funds disbursed throughout the year under a letter-of-credit arrangement whereby the plans draw down funds in their accounts as claims are paid.

OPM maintains in the U.S. Treasury contingency reserve funds for community-rated plans,[51] and may charge up to 3% of a plan's premium to establish and maintain the fund. However, unlike that for experience-rated plans, the contingency reserve fund for community-rated plans can be used only by OPM (not the plan) if OPM approves an adjustment during a "reconciliation" process that usually takes place in the month of March. For instance, HMOs generally estimate their rates in the spring and negotiate their contracts with OPM in August. The plan year begins the following January. If there are changes in the program or in the community benefit package between the time the plan estimated the rates and implementation of the plan in January, OPM reconciles those changes with the previously established premiums and negotiates an adjustment. (OPM allows adjustment only for specified reasons, excluding a plan's underestimate of costs based on group demographics.) Because payments to HMOs are not based on claims, the government does not use the letter-of-credit draw-down approach to disburse funds to the plans, but pays the plans specified amounts in installments throughout the year.

OPM's Role with Setting Profits

The "service charge" (profit) paid to fee-for-service plans by OPM is calculated according to detailed regulations.[52] There is no guaranteed minimum amount, but the maximum is 1.1% of projected incurred claims and administrative costs. OPM contract officers monitor plan performance throughout a plan year and maintain data which are used to evaluate plan performance and determine profit. Profit is based on six factors: (1) contractor performance regarding such responsibilities as accurate and timely claims processing, handling of claims disputes, and general beneficial innovations; (2) contract cost risk factors, including group size (smaller enrollments receive credit for higher risk), and certain demographics and the plan's willingness to assume risk; (3) federal socioeconomic programs, such as programs to deter drug abuse by considering the quality of the contractor's policies and procedures and the extent of unusual effort or achievement demonstrated; (4) capital investments (this is a general federal acquisition factor but seldom applicable under FEHBP); (5) cost control, such as contractor-initiated efforts to improve benefit design, cost-sharing, or innovative peer review procedures; and (6) independent development of administrative systems that improve cost efficiency and for which the contractor assumed the development costs.

Each of these profit factors is scored with regard to the plan's performance in the previous year, and the sum of the scores determines the profit percentage. The "profit" margins for FEHBP fee-for-service plans are not large, but the plans in the program experience little risk because they may make up losses experienced in the past year through increases in premiums in the following year (or they may draw down surplus contingency reserves). Plan income in excess of that which

---

[51] Community-rated plans are basically the local HMOs, whose payment is based on comparable rates offered to other plans in the community. Additionally, these plans may negotiate upgrades and/or required services. The profit for community-rated plans may be larger than experience-rated plans, as well as the risk.

[52] 48 CFR §1615.4.

had been estimated when premiums were set for a given year may be carried forward and used to limit premium increases in the following year.

For the community-rated plans, OPM negotiates with the HMO plans to receive a capitated payment for each federal enrollee. The payment amount is based on comparable rates offered to other plans in the community, plus negotiated upgrades to the community benefit package. HMOs may compute their community rate using factors such as age and sex. During a reconciliation process at the end of the contract year, OPM determines the appropriateness of the capitated payments to each HMO, and settles with the HMOs accordingly. The profit rate HMOs receive based on the community rate may be larger than that available to fee-for-service plans under FEHBP.

Financing OPM's Costs for Administering FEHBP

The only administrative costs of the federal government for FEHBP that can be identified explicitly are the costs of OPM's headquarters staff. For 2009, OPM employed about 191 FTEs who are responsible for FEHBP.[53] This staff includes the actuaries and employees who negotiate with carriers, monitor plans and contracts, and generally oversee all aspects of program administration. OPM adds a charge to each plan's premium, limited to 1% of the premium, to cover these administrative costs.[54] Generally the charge is less than 1%. There is no separate accounting for the costs associated with agency personnel who carry out administrative tasks associated with FEHBP as well as the other pay and benefit programs for federal workers. Plan carriers' administrative costs are included in their premiums. To the extent that plans compete for enrollees on basis of premiums, they have an incentive for administrative efficiency. However, OPM does not ask for detailed administrative cost data, although it periodically audits certain overhead charges.

Other Administrative Roles/Activities

Data Warehousing: OPM is creating a new health information management system that will, among other things, be used to collect, manage, and analyze health services data for FEHBP.[55] Generally, OPM analysts will use the de-identified data for such analytic purposes as the examination of health trends, development of risk adjustment methodologies, and oversight of pharmacy pricing and negotiation. Data with personal identifiers may also be used within OPM,[56] in accordance with applicable privacy standards, for the purposes of a congressional inquiry, for judicial and administrative proceedings, and for investigations by law enforcement officials.[57]

---

[53] The 2009 estimate of FTEs is most recent publicly-available estimate. FY2010, Office of Personnel Management Congressional Budget Justification Performance Budget.

[54] 5 CFR §890.503.

[55] 75 *Federal Register* 61532, October 5, 2010; 76 *Federal Register* 35050, June 15, 2011.

[56] Only de-identified data will be released outside of OPM.

[57] Under the privacy rule of the Health Insurance Portability and Accountability Act (HIPAA, P.L. 104-191), identifiable information refers to data that are explicitly linked to a particular individual and data items that reasonably could be expected to allow individual identification. Potential identifiers include, but are not limited to, name and social security number; voice and fax telephone numbers; electronic mail addresses; medical record numbers, health plan beneficiary numbers, or other health plan account numbers; biometric identifiers, including finger and voice prints; and full face photographic images.

Grievance and Appeals: All plan brochures include an explanation of the procedures enrollees should follow if they disagree with a denial of coverage or payment. An enrollee must first submit a written request to the plan for reconsideration within six months of the denial of coverage. Within 30 days of receiving the request, the plan must approve the claim, request additional information or provide a written statement explaining the denial.[58]

If the plan decides against the enrollee, a written appeal can be filed with OPM within 90 days of the plan's second denial. If OPM determines the enrollee is entitled to coverage, the plan must provide or pay for the care. If OPM decides against the enrollee, he or she can appeal in federal district court.

Sanctions: OPM may, and in some cases must, apply sanctions to health care providers.[59] These sanctions include debarment, suspension, civil monetary penalties, and financial assessments. The regulations establish the circumstances under which these sanctions may occur, along with procedures for appeals.

State Law Exemptions: The terms of a contract relating to coverage or benefits, including payments, supersede and preempt any state or local laws and regulations relating to health insurance or plans. While OPM requires HMOs to provide their FEHBP plan enrollees with mandated state benefits, OPM has the authority to override these requirements.

---

[58] 5 CFR §890.105.

[59] 5 CFR §890.1001.

Appendix B. The United States Postal Service and FEHBP

Similar to most other federal agencies, the United States Postal Service (USPS)[60] offers health care benefits to its employees and annuitants through FEHBP; however, as an agency, the USPS is governed by arrangements that are unique within the federal government in regard to contributing to health care benefits for its employees and annuitants.

USPS employees have collective bargaining rights, including for compensation and benefits. The Postal Reorganization Act (PRA, P.L. 91-375) gives USPS employees these rights and requires that "fringe benefits," including health insurance, offered to employees are at least as favorable as the fringe benefits that were in effect when PRA was enacted (1970). A result of these provisions is that unlike other federal agencies whose contribution to their employees' and annuitants' premiums are determined by a formula set in law,[61] the USPS contribution to employees' premiums is determined through collective bargaining agreements.[62]

Historically, the USPS has paid a larger share of employees' health insurance premiums compared to other federal agencies. On average, the USPS paid 79% of postal employees' premiums, while other federal agencies paid 71% of employees' premiums.[63] According to a recent GAO report, the USPS contribution rates will decrease in coming years under current agreements with its unions and management associations. Under the current collective bargaining agreements and arbitration awards, the USPS contribution for health care premiums for employees covered by collective bargaining will decrease to approximately 76% in 2016.[64]

In most federal agencies, the government contribution to health benefits for its annuitants is not paid by the agency, but from annual appropriations;[65] however, the Consolidated Omnibus Budget Reconciliation Act (COBRA, P.L. 99-272) requires that the USPS pay the government's share of health benefits for its annuitants. Additionally, the Postal Accountability and Enhancement Act (PAEA, P.L. 109-435) creates a prefunding obligation for the USPS for its annuitant health care costs. PAEA requires the USPS to pay more than $5 billion annually from FY2007 to FY2016 to build a fund from which annuitants and employees will be paid come FY2017.

---

[60] While still a federal agency, 39 U.S.C. 201 declares the USPS to be an "independent establishment of the executive branch."

[61] For an explanation of how the split between employee and employer contribution for premiums is determined in FEHBP, see "Premiums" in this report.

[62] For annuitant coverage, the USPS contribution to premiums is the same as it is in other federal agencies.

[63] CRS analysis of OPM data.

[64] U.S. Government Accountability Office. U.S. Postal Service: Proposed Health Plan Could Improve Financial Condition, but Impact on Medicare and Other Issues Should Be Weighed before Approval, GAO-13-658, July 2013, http://gao.gov/assets/660/656011.pdf.

[65] Title 5 §8906(g)(1).

Author Contact Information

Annie L. Mach
Analyst in Health Care Financing
amach@crs.loc.gov, 7-7825

Ada S. Cornell
Information Research Specialist
acornell@crs.loc.gov, 7-3742